Essential Oils

The 7-Day Plan to Melt Away Stress, Boost Your Energy, and Thrive in Your Busy Life

Scarlett Savage

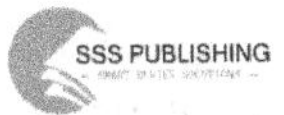

SSS PUBLISHING

Contents

Introduction: A Wake-Up Call for High-Achieving Women

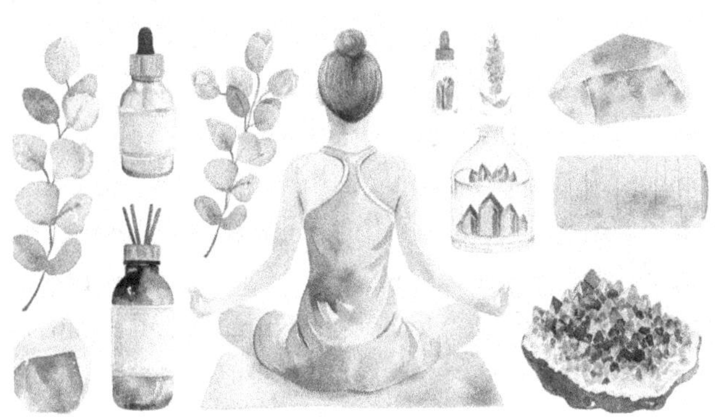

You know that feeling when you're running on empty, but you keep pushing through because there's just so much to do? That constant sense of overwhelm, the nagging guilt that you're not doing enough, and the fear that if you slow down, everything will come crashing down? If you're a high-achieving woman juggling multiple responsibilities, I bet you know exactly what I'm talking about.

Hi, I'm Scarlett Savage, and I've been there too. As a busy entrepreneur, wife, and mother, I've experienced firsthand the toll that chronic stress can take on our minds, bodies, and spirits. I've struggled with burnout, anxiety, and the feeling that I was constantly falling short, no matter how hard I tried.

But here's the thing: it doesn't have to be this way. We don't have to accept stress and overwhelm as the price of success. There is another path – one that allows us to thrive, not just survive, as we pursue our dreams and care for the people we love.

That's why I've written this book. Because I believe that every high-achieving woman deserves to have the tools and strategies she needs to manage stress, prioritize self-care, and live a life that feels balanced, fulfilling, and joyful.

If you're feeling overwhelmed by stress and looking to take back control of your well-being, you've come to the right place. In the following pages, I'll introduce you to a groundbreaking technique for managing stress that has made a huge difference in my life and for many other women. It's called the **Sensory Shift Method**, and it uses the power of essential oils and aromatherapy to help you change your mindset, increase your energy, and find a sense of peace and balance – even when things get hectic.

Let's pause for a second and really think about the stress that's weighing down a lot of successful women out there. You should know, you're definitely not the only one dealing with this. Now, let's talk about the Sensory Shift Method and what it's all about.

In fact, research shows that women are twice as likely as men to experience symptoms of stress and burnout. We're more likely to report feeling overwhelmed, exhausted, and emotionally drained, and we're also more likely to neglect our own self-care in the process.

There are a lot of factors contributing to this stress epidemic among high-achieving women. For one, we're often juggling multiple roles and responsibilities – from our careers to our families to our communities – and the pressure to excel in all of these areas can be intense. We're also more likely to internalize stress and blame ourselves when things don't go perfectly, rather than recognizing that stress is a natural response to the demands of modern life.

But here's the good news: while we may not be able to eliminate stress from our lives completely, we can learn to manage it in a way that allows us to thrive. And that's exactly what the Sensory Shift Method is all about.

At its core, the Sensory Shift Method is about harnessing the power of our senses – particularly our sense of smell – to quickly shift our mindset and emotional state. You see, our sense of smell is uniquely connected to the parts of our brain that process emotion and memory. When we inhale an essential oil, the scent molecules travel directly to the limbic system, which is responsible for regulating our stress response, our mood, and our overall sense of well-being.

This means that by simply inhaling a specific blend of essential oils, we can quickly calm our nervous system, reduce feelings of anxiety and overwhelm, and promote a sense of balance and resilience. And when we combine this with simple mindset techniques and self-care practices, the impact is even more powerful.

In the chapters ahead, I'll guide you through the science behind the Sensory Shift Method, and I'll share with you specific essential oil blends and rituals that you can use to manage stress in the moment, promote restful sleep, boost your energy and focus, and so much more.

But I want to be clear: this isn't just about quick fixes or band-aid solutions. The Sensory Shift Method is about creating lasting transformation in the way you relate to stress and care for yourself. It's about shifting your mindset, your habits, and your overall approach to well-being, so that you can thrive in all areas of your life.

And the best part? It doesn't require a lot of time, money, or special equipment. The Sensory Shift Method is designed to be simple, accessible, and easy to integrate into even the busiest of schedules. All you need is a few key essential oils, a willingness to experiment with new rituals and practices, and a commitment to prioritizing your own well-being.

Are you ready to take control of your stress levels, reclaim your energy and vitality, and step into a life of greater balance, purpose, and joy? If so, I welcome you to join me on this journey. In the pages ahead, you'll find a powerful roadmap for transformation that has the potential to not only change your relationship with stress, but also your entire life.

Let's get started, shall we?

Chapter 1

Understanding the Stress Epidemic and Its Impact on High-Achieving Women

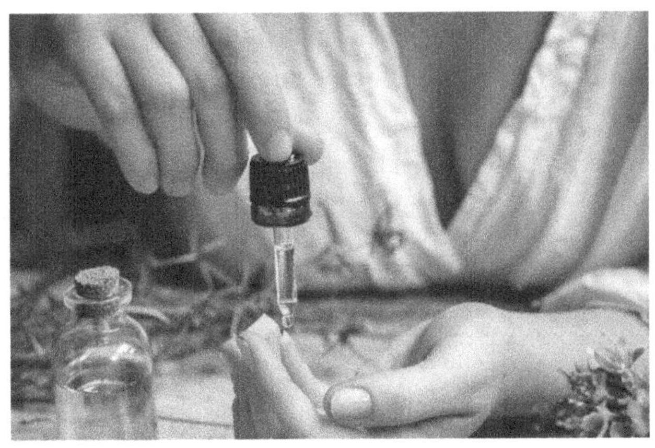

The Hidden Toll of Chronic Stress on Mind, Body, and Spirit

Close your eyes and imagine this: you're a high-achieving woman, juggling a demanding career, family responsibilities, and personal goals. You're constantly on the go, pushing yourself to excel in every area of your life. But beneath the surface of your success, there's a silent struggle taking place – the toll of chronic stress on your mind, body, and spirit.

You're not alone in this struggle. In fact, chronic stress has become an epidemic among high-achieving women, with far-reaching consequences that often go unrecognized or unaddressed. But here's the truth: we can no longer afford to ignore the impact of stress on our well-being.

When we talk about the toll of chronic stress, we're referring to the cumulative effects of living in a constant state of fight-or-flight. This happens when our bodies are repeatedly exposed to stressors – whether it's a looming deadline, a difficult conversation, or the pressure to be everything to everyone – without adequate time to rest and recover.

Over time, this chronic activation of the stress response can lead to a wide range of physical, emotional, and mental health consequences. Let's take a closer look at each of these areas:

Physical Health Consequences:

One of the most noticeable ways that chronic stress takes a toll on our bodies is through physical symptoms. When we're stressed, our bodies release a flood of hormones like cortisol and adrenaline, which can lead to:

- Headaches and migraines: The tension and muscle contractions caused by stress can trigger headaches and migraines, making it difficult to focus and function.
- Muscle tension and pain: Chronic stress can cause our muscles to remain in a constant state of tension, leading to pain, stiffness, and reduced mobility.
- Digestive issues: Stress can disrupt the delicate balance of our digestive system, causing symptoms like acid reflux, bloating, constipation, and irritable bowel syndrome.
- Weakened immune function: When our bodies are in a constant state of stress, our immune system can become

compromised, making us more susceptible to illness and disease.

- Cardiovascular problems: Chronic stress can contribute to high blood pressure, increased heart rate, and inflammation, all of which can increase the risk of heart attack and stroke.
- Hormonal imbalances: Stress can disrupt the delicate balance of our hormones, leading to issues like irregular menstrual cycles, fertility problems, and other reproductive health concerns.

These physical symptoms are our bodies' way of telling us that something is out of balance – that we're pushing ourselves too hard and not giving ourselves the rest and care we need. But all too often, we ignore these warning signs, pushing through the pain and discomfort in the name of productivity and achievement.

Emotional Health Consequences:

In addition to the physical toll of chronic stress, there's also a significant emotional impact. When we're chronically stressed, we may experience:

- Anxiety and worry: Chronic stress can cause feelings of anxiety and worry to become constant and overwhelming, making it difficult to relax and enjoy life.
- Irritability and mood swings: Stress can make us more reactive and sensitive to triggers, leading to mood swings and irritability that strain our relationships and daily interactions.
- Depression and feelings of hopelessness: Over time, chronic stress can contribute to feelings of depression, hopelessness, and helplessness, making it difficult to find joy and purpose in life.
- Difficulty concentrating and making decisions: When our minds are consumed with stress and worry, it can be

challenging to focus on tasks and make clear, confident decisions.

- A sense of disconnection or isolation: Stress can cause us to withdraw from others and feel disconnected or isolated, even when we're surrounded by people who care about us.

These emotional symptoms can be particularly challenging for high-achieving women, who often feel pressure to maintain a façade of strength and competence, even when they're struggling internally. We may feel like we can't afford to show vulnerability or ask for help, for fear of being seen as weak or incapable.

Mental Health Consequences:

Finally, chronic stress can take a significant toll on our mental health and cognitive function. When we're in a constant state of fight-or-flight, our brains are flooded with stress hormones that can impair our ability to:

- Focus and concentrate on tasks: Chronic stress can make it difficult to maintain focus and attention, leading to decreased productivity and performance.
- Remember important information and details: Stress can impair our memory and recall, causing us to forget important details and struggle with tasks that once came easily.
- Think creatively and come up with new ideas: When our minds are consumed with stress and worry, it can be challenging to think outside the box and generate innovative solutions.
- Process and regulate our emotions effectively: Chronic stress can make it difficult to process and regulate our emotions in healthy ways, leading to emotional reactivity and instability.

- Make sound decisions and judgments: Stress can cloud our judgment and decision-making abilities, causing us to make impulsive or irrational choices.

Over time, this chronic exposure to stress can even lead to changes in the structure and function of our brains, increasing our risk of developing conditions like anxiety disorders, depression, and cognitive decline.

The Invisible Impact on our Spirit:

But perhaps the most insidious toll of chronic stress is the way it can erode our sense of self, our purpose, and our overall spiritual well-being. When we're constantly running on empty, juggling too many demands and responsibilities, it's easy to lose sight of what really matters to us – our values, our passions, and our authentic selves.

We may feel like we're just going through the motions, disconnected from the things that once brought us joy and fulfillment. We may start to doubt our own abilities and self-worth, feeling like we're never enough, no matter how much we achieve.

This erosion of our spirit can be subtle and gradual, but its impact is profound. It can leave us feeling depleted, unfulfilled, and questioning the very purpose and meaning of our lives.

But here's the good news: we don't have to accept this toll of chronic stress as inevitable. We have the power to take control of our well-being, to prioritize our own self-care, and to cultivate a sense of resilience and purpose in the face of life's challenges.

It starts with recognizing the hidden impact of stress on our minds, bodies, and spirits – and making a commitment to do something about it. It means learning to tune into our own needs and desires, setting boundaries to protect our time and energy, and investing in practices that nourish and sustain us from the inside out.

And that's exactly what the rest of this book is all about. In the chapters ahead, we'll explore a revolutionary approach to stress management that combines the power of essential oils, mindset shifts, and simple self-care practices to help you reclaim your well-being and thrive in all areas of your life.

if you're tired of dealing with chronic stress and want to live a more balanced, purposeful, and joyful life, then keep reading. The path to better stress management begins here.

The Myth of Work-Life Balance and the Importance of Self-Care

As high-achieving women, we've been sold the idea that we can have it all – a thriving career, a loving family, a fulfilling personal life – if we just work hard enough and find the perfect balance. But here's the truth: the concept of "work-life balance" is a myth, and chasing after it can actually contribute to the cycle of chronic stress and burnout.

The reality is that life is messy, unpredictable, and full of competing demands. There will always be times when one area of our lives requires more attention than others, and that's okay. The key is not to strive for some elusive sense of perfect balance, but rather to cultivate a sense of harmony and integration among the different facets of our lives.

And that's where self-care comes in. Self-care is not a luxury or an indulgence – it's a necessary practice for maintaining our physical, emotional, and mental well-being. When we prioritize self-care, we're better equipped to handle the inevitable ups and downs of life, and to show up as our best selves in all areas of our lives.

But for many high-achieving women, self-care can feel like just another item on our already overwhelming to-do list. We may feel guilty for taking time for ourselves, or worry that we're being selfish or unproductive. We may also struggle with the idea of putting our own needs first, especially when we're so used to taking care of everyone else.

However, the truth is that self-care is not selfish – it's essential. When we neglect our own needs and well-being, we're not only hurting ourselves, but also diminishing our ability to be there for the people and things that matter most to us. We cannot pour from an empty cup, and self-care is how we fill ourselves back up.

So what does self-care look like in practice? It can take many different forms, depending on our individual needs and preferences. Some examples might include:

- Getting enough sleep and rest
- Nourishing our bodies with healthy food and movement
- Taking breaks throughout the day to stretch, breathe, and recharge
- Engaging in activities that bring us joy and fulfillment, like hobbies or creative pursuits
- Connecting with loved ones and cultivating supportive relationships
- Seeking professional help when needed, such as therapy or coaching
- Practicing mindfulness and stress-reduction techniques, like meditation or deep breathing

The key is to approach self-care not as another chore or obligation, but as an act of self-love and self-preservation. It's about tuning into our own needs and desires, and making a commitment to prioritize our well-being, even in the face of life's demands and challenges.

Of course, this is easier said than done. Many of us have deeply ingrained beliefs and patterns around self-care and self-worth, and it can take time and practice to shift these habits. We may also face practical barriers to self-care, such as lack of time, resources, or support.

That's why it's so important to approach self-care with compassion and flexibility. It's not about perfection or doing everything "right" – it's about making small, consistent choices that add up over time to support our overall well-being.

And that's where the Sensory Shift Method comes in. By harnessing the power of essential oils and aromatherapy, we can quickly and easily incorporate moments of self-care into our daily lives, even when we're short on time or energy. The simple act of inhaling a calming or uplifting scent can help us shift our mindset, release tension, and reconnect with ourselves, even in the midst of a busy day.

In the coming chapters, we'll explore the science behind aromatherapy and the Sensory Shift Method, and provide practical guidance on how to use essential oils to support your self-care practice. But for now, I invite you to simply begin by noticing your own relationship to self-care, and considering how you might start to prioritize your own needs and well-being, one small step at a time.

The Power of Natural Solutions: Introducing Essential Oils and Aromatherapy

You might be curious about how essential oils and aromatherapy fit into the whole picture of dealing with the wear and tear that constant stress has on our mental, physical, and emotional well-being, especially since we've talked about how crucial self-care is in handling that stress.

The answer is: a powerful one. Essential oils and aromatherapy have been used for centuries in traditional healing practices around the world, and in recent years, modern science has begun to catch up, providing evidence for their remarkable therapeutic benefits.

At their core, essential oils are highly concentrated plant extracts that capture the natural essence and healing properties of the plant. They're typically extracted through a process of steam distillation or cold pressing, which preserves the volatile compounds that give each oil its unique aroma and therapeutic qualities.

When we inhale the aroma of an essential oil, those volatile compounds enter our bloodstream and interact with our body's systems in a variety of ways. Some oils have a calming and relaxing effect on the nervous system, helping to reduce stress and anxiety. Others have an uplifting and energizing effect, helping to boost mood and mental clarity. Still others have anti-inflammatory, analgesic, or immune-supportive properties, helping to promote physical healing and resilience.

But the power of essential oils goes beyond just their physiological effects. There's also a profound psychological and emotional component to aromatherapy, one that ties into the intimate connection between our sense of smell and our limbic system, the part of our brain that processes emotion and memory.

When we inhale an aroma, it triggers an immediate response in the limbic system, bypassing the conscious mind and directly influencing our emotional state. This is why certain scents can instantly transport us back to a cherished memory, or why the aroma of fresh-baked bread can make us feel warm and comforted.

In the context of stress management and self-care, this emotional component of aromatherapy is particularly powerful. By intentionally using essential oils to shift our emotional state, we can quickly and easily access a sense of calm, balance, and well-being, even in the face of life's challenges.

And this is where the concept of the Sensory Shift Method comes in. Developed by aromatherapist and self-care expert Jessie Cole, the Sensory Shift Method is a simple yet powerful approach to using essential oils for stress relief and emotional balance.

At its core, the Sensory Shift Method involves using specific essential oil blends to promote three key emotional states: calm, clarity, and resilience. By inhaling these blends at strategic points throughout the day, we can quickly shift our mindset and emotional state, promoting a sense of grounding, focus, and inner strength.

But the Sensory Shift Method is more than just a set of essential oil blends — it's a comprehensive approach to self-care that integrates mindfulness, self-reflection, and practical stress-management techniques. Through a series of simple yet powerful rituals and practices, the Sensory Shift Method helps us cultivate a deeper sense of self-awareness, self-compassion, and emotional resilience.

In the next few sections, we're going to explore the Sensory Shift

Method in detail. I'll walk you through how you can use essential oils and aromatherapy to change how you handle stress and find a better sense of peace and wellness..

But for now, I invite you to simply begin by exploring the power of scent in your own life. Take a moment to notice the aromas around you – the fresh smell of coffee in the morning, the sweet fragrance of a blooming flower, the comforting scent of a loved one's perfume.

Notice how those scents make you feel, and consider how you might start to use scent intentionally to shift your emotional state and promote a sense of calm and balance. Perhaps you might light a scented candle during your evening wind-down routine, or keep a small bottle of lavender oil on your desk to help you stay grounded during a busy workday.

Remember, the power of natural solutions like essential oils and aromatherapy lies not just in their physiological effects, but in their ability to help us connect with ourselves on a deeper level – to tune into our own needs and desires, and to cultivate a greater sense of self-awareness and self-care.

Let's explore the Sensory Shift Method together and see how essential oils can really make a difference. I want you to be curious, open, and kind to yourself as we go through this. Believe that you've got what it takes to handle life's ups and downs. With the right tools and a bit of help, you can find more balance, meaning, and happiness in your life, just by taking it one breath at a time.

Chapter 2

The Science of Scent: How Essential Oils Work to Reduce Stress and Promote Balance

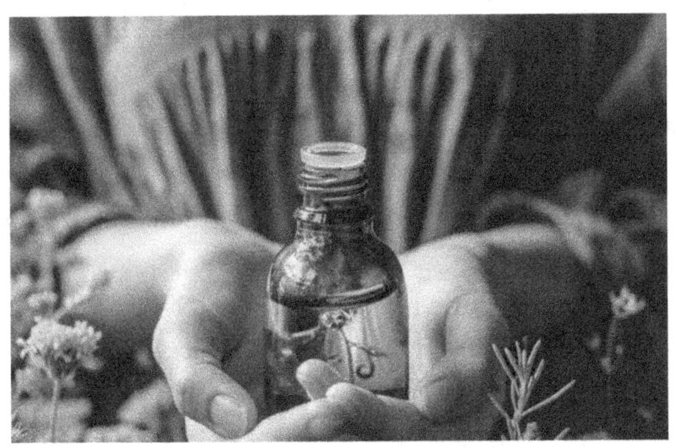

The Olfactory System: The Direct Link Between Scent and Emotion

Have you ever wondered why certain scents can instantly transport you back to a cherished memory or evoke a specific emotion? The answer lies in the fascinating connection between our sense of smell and our emotional processing center in the brain.

11

To understand how essential oils can have such a powerful impact on our stress levels and overall well-being, it's important to first explore the science behind our sense of smell, or the olfactory system.

The olfactory system is one of the most ancient and primitive sensory systems in the human body, evolving over millions of years to help us navigate our environment, find food, and avoid danger. Unlike our other senses, which are routed through the thalamus before reaching the cerebral cortex, the olfactory system has a direct link to the limbic system, the part of our brain responsible for processing emotions and memories.

When we inhale a scent, whether it's from an essential oil, a freshly baked cookie, or a blooming rose, the odor molecules travel up the nasal cavity and bind to specialized receptors in the olfactory epithelium. This triggers a complex cascade of neural activity, sending signals directly to the limbic system and activating the amygdala, hippocampus, and other brain regions involved in emotional processing and memory formation.

The amygdala, in particular, plays a crucial role in our emotional response to scent. This almond-shaped structure, located deep within the temporal lobe, is responsible for processing and regulating emotions, particularly those related to fear, anxiety, and stress. When we inhale a calming scent like lavender or chamomile, it can help to soothe an overactive amygdala, reducing feelings of anxiety and promoting a sense of relaxation.

Similarly, the hippocampus, which is involved in forming and storing memories, is highly responsive to scent. This is why certain aromas can instantly evoke vivid memories and emotions from the past, whether it's the comforting smell of a loved one's perfume or the nostalgic scent of a favorite childhood food.

But the olfactory system's impact on our emotions and memories goes beyond just the individual level – it's also deeply intertwined with our social and cultural experiences. In many cultures around the world, scent plays a central role in ritual, celebration, and healing practices, from the use of incense in religious ceremonies to the application of aromatic oils in traditional medicine.

Our emotional associations with scent are shaped by these cultural and personal experiences, as well as by our individual biology and genetics. Some people may find the scent of peppermint invigorating and energizing, while others may find it overpowering or unpleasant. Similarly, a scent that evokes positive memories for one person may trigger negative emotions for another, based on their unique life experiences.

This complex interplay between scent, emotion, and memory is what makes aromatherapy such a powerful tool for promoting emotional well-being and resilience. By intentionally using essential oils to stimulate the olfactory system and activate specific brain regions, we can harness the power of scent to shift our mood, release tension, and cultivate a greater sense of calm and balance.

Aromatherapy does more than just make us feel good mentally. It actually has a physical impact on our bodies too. Essential oils are packed with chemicals that can do things like lessen swelling, ease pain, or help our immune system fight off bugs.

For example, the essential oil of peppermint contains menthol, a compound that has been shown to have analgesic and anti-inflammatory properties, making it useful for relieving headaches and soothing sore muscles. Similarly, the essential oil of tea tree contains terpinen-4-ol, a compound with powerful antimicrobial properties that can help to fight off harmful bacteria and viruses.

But while the physiological effects of essential oils are certainly important, it's the olfactory system's direct link to our emotions and memories that makes aromatherapy such a powerful tool for stress management and self-care. By tapping into this primal sensory system, we can quickly and easily shift our emotional state, releasing tension and cultivating a greater sense of calm, clarity, and resilience.

The Chemistry of Essential Oils: Terpenes, Phenols, and Esters

While the olfactory system's direct link to our emotions and memories is a crucial component of aromatherapy's power, it's not the only factor at play. The unique chemical composition of each essential oil also contributes to its therapeutic effects on the mind and body.

Essential oils are highly concentrated plant extracts that contain a complex mixture of chemical compounds, each with its own unique properties and potential benefits. These compounds can be broadly divided into several categories, including terpenes, phenols, and esters.

Terpenes are the most common class of compounds found in essential oils, and they play a key role in the plants' natural defense systems against pests and disease. Terpenes are responsible for the distinctive aromas of many essential oils, such as the fresh, clean scent of lemon or the warm, woody aroma of cedarwood.

But terpenes are more than just pleasant fragrances – they also have a wide range of therapeutic properties that can benefit our physical and emotional well-being. For example, limonene, a terpene found in citrus oils like lemon and orange, has been shown to have antidepressant and anxiolytic (anxiety-reducing) effects, as well as potential anti-cancer properties.

Similarly, pinene, a terpene found in pine and other coniferous oils, has been shown to have anti-inflammatory and bronchodilatory effects, making it useful for respiratory issues like asthma and allergies. And linalool, a terpene found in lavender and other floral oils, has been shown to have sedative and stress-reducing effects, making it a popular choice for promoting relaxation and sleep.

Phenols are another important class of compounds found in essential oils, known for their strong antioxidant and antimicrobial properties. Oils high in phenols, such as clove, thyme, and oregano, are often used for their cleansing and purifying effects, as well as for boosting immune function and fighting off harmful bacteria and viruses.

Eugenol, a phenol found in clove oil, has been shown to have potent analgesic and anti-inflammatory effects, making it useful for relieving pain and soothing sore muscles and joints. Thymol, a phenol found in thyme oil, has powerful antimicrobial properties that can help to fight off infections and support respiratory health.

Esters are a third class of compounds found in essential oils, known for their soothing and balancing effects on the mind and body. Oils high in esters, such as lavender, bergamot, and ylang-ylang, are often used for their calming and uplifting properties, as well as for promoting skin health and reducing inflammation.

Linalyl acetate, an ester found in lavender and bergamot oils, has been shown to have sedative and anxiolytic effects, making it useful for reducing stress and promoting relaxation. Geranyl acetate, an ester found in rose and geranium oils, has been shown to have balancing and harmonizing effects on the emotions, as well as potential benefits for hormone regulation and skin health.

Of course, these are just a few examples of the many chemical compounds found in essential oils, and the potential therapeutic benefits they offer. Each essential oil contains a unique blend of these compounds, which work synergistically to create its distinct aroma and therapeutic profile.

It's important to note that the quality and purity of an essential oil can greatly impact its chemical composition and therapeutic effectiveness. Poor quality or adulterated oils may contain synthetic fragrances, fillers, or other contaminants that can dilute or alter the oil's natural chemistry, reducing its potential benefits and even posing safety risks.

That's why it's crucial to choose high-quality, pure essential oils from reputable sources, and to use them safely and responsibly under the guidance of a qualified aromatherapist or healthcare provider. When used properly, however, the chemical complexity of essential oils can be a powerful ally in supporting our physical, emotional, and mental well-being.

The Evidence-Based Benefits of Aromatherapy for Stress Management

While the therapeutic use of essential oils and aromatherapy has a long and rich history in traditional healing practices around the world, modern science is now beginning to catch up, providing evidence-based support for their effectiveness in reducing stress and promoting relaxation.

Numerous studies have explored the impact of aromatherapy on stress and anxiety levels, using a variety of essential oils and application methods. While the specific results may vary depending on the oil used and the individual's unique biology and experiences, the overall trend is clear: aromatherapy can be a powerful tool for promoting calm, reducing tension, and supporting emotional well-being.

One of the most well-studied essential oils for stress relief is lavender, which has been shown to have significant anxiolytic and sedative effects. A 2012 study published in the Journal of Alternative and Complementary Medicine found that inhaling lavender oil for just five minutes was effective in reducing stress and anxiety levels in dental patients waiting for treatment.

Similarly, a 2013 study published in the journal Evidence-Based Complementary and Alternative Medicine found that lavender aromatherapy was effective in reducing stress and improving sleep quality in intensive care unit patients. The study participants who received lavender aromatherapy reported significantly lower levels of stress and anxiety, as well as better sleep quality, compared to those who did not receive aromatherapy.

Other essential oils that have been shown to have stress-reducing effects include bergamot, which has been found to lower cortisol levels and promote relaxation; frankincense, which has been shown to reduce anxiety and depression symptoms; and ylang-ylang, which has been found to lower blood pressure and heart rate, indicating a calming effect on the nervous system.

But the benefits of aromatherapy for stress management go beyond just the physiological effects of the essential oils themselves. The act of taking time to engage in an aromatherapy practice, whether it's through inhalation, massage, or other application methods, can also be a powerful form of self-care and mindfulness.

By intentionally setting aside time to focus on our own well-being, we send a powerful message to ourselves that we are worthy of care and attention. The simple act of inhaling a calming scent or applying a soothing oil to our skin can be a reminder to slow down, breathe deeply, and tune into our own needs and desires.

Moreover, the use of aromatherapy can be a powerful tool for promoting a sense of ritual and routine in our self-care practices. By incorporating specific essential oils or blends into our daily routines, such as a morning energizing blend or an evening relaxation ritual, we can create a sense of structure and predictability that can be grounding and reassuring in times of stress.

Absolutely, aromatherapy can be a great way to help you chill out, but remember, it's not the be-all and end-all. Essential oils are awesome for giving your mood a little boost, but they're not going to fix everything. If you're really feeling the pressure, it's super important to talk to a pro and make sure you're living a healthy life. Plus, there are tons of other ways to cut down on stress that have solid proof behind them. So, think of aromatherapy as your chill-out buddy, not your sole stress-buster.

But when used in conjunction with other self-care practices, such as regular exercise, healthy eating, and mindfulness meditation, aromatherapy can be a valuable addition to our stress management arsenal. By tapping into the power of scent to shift our mood, release tension, and promote relaxation, we can cultivate a greater sense of resilience and inner peace, even in the face of life's challenges.

Chapter 3

The Sensory Shift Method: A Revolutionary Approach to Stress Relief

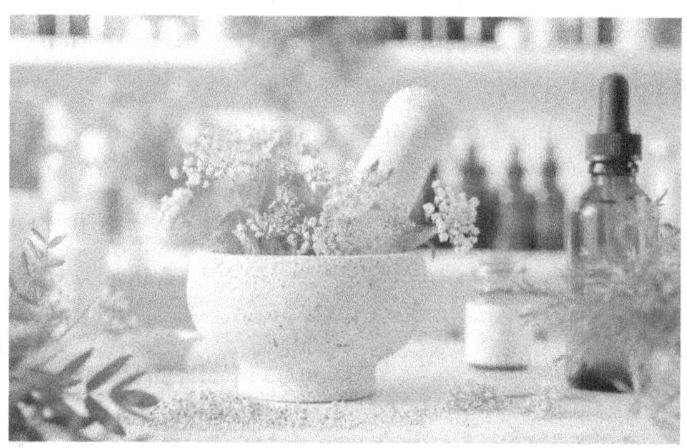

Have you ever found yourself in a situation where stress seemed to be taking over your life, leaving you feeling overwhelmed, exhausted, and on the brink of burnout? If so, you're not alone. In today's fast-paced, high-pressure world, stress has become an all-too-common experience for many of us, particularly for high-achieving women juggling multiple roles and responsibilities.

But what if I told you that there was a simple, yet powerful way

18

to transform your relationship with stress, using nothing more than the power of your own senses? Enter the Sensory Shift Method: a revolutionary approach to stress relief that combines the science of aromatherapy with the art of mindfulness and self-care.

At its core, the Sensory Shift Method is based on the idea that our senses, particularly our sense of smell, have a direct and powerful impact on our emotional state. By harnessing the power of scent through the use of essential oils, we can quickly and effectively shift our mood, release tension, and promote a sense of calm and balance.

But the Sensory Shift Method is more than just a collection of pleasant fragrances – it's a comprehensive system for stress management that incorporates three key pillars: scent, mindset, and self-care. Let's take a closer look at each of these pillars and how they work together to create a powerful tool for stress relief.

The Three Pillars of the Sensory Shift Method: Scent, Mindset, and Self-Care

The first pillar of the Sensory Shift Method is scent, which we've already explored in some depth in the previous chapter. By using specific essential oils or blends that have been shown to have calming, uplifting, or balancing effects, we can harness the power of aromatherapy to quickly shift our emotional state and promote relaxation.

But scent alone is not enough to create lasting change in our relationship with stress. That's where the second pillar of the Sensory Shift Method comes in: mindset. Our thoughts and beliefs about stress, and our ability to cope with it, play a huge role in how we experience and respond to stressful situations.

By cultivating a mindset of resilience, self-compassion, and growth, we can begin to reframe stress as an opportunity for learning and personal development, rather than as a threat to be avoided or eliminated. This shift in perspective can be incredibly empowering, allowing us to approach challenges with greater confidence and adaptability.

But cultivating a resilient mindset is not always easy, especially when we're in the midst of a stressful situation. That's where the power of scent comes in – by using specific essential oils or blends that promote feelings of calm, clarity, and groundedness, we can create a sensory anchor that helps us access a more positive and empowered state of mind.

For example, when we're feeling overwhelmed or anxious, we might use a grounding blend of essential oils that includes earthy scents like vetiver, frankincense, and cedarwood. These scents can help us feel more rooted and centered, allowing us to approach the situation with greater clarity and perspective.

Or, when we're feeling mentally fatigued or stuck, we might use an uplifting blend that includes invigorating scents like peppermint, rosemary, and lemon. These scents can help to clear mental fog, boost focus and concentration, and inspire creative problem-solving.

The third pillar of the Sensory Shift Method is self-care, which is essential for managing stress and promoting overall well-being. When we're stressed, it's all too easy to neglect our own needs and prioritize others' demands over our own self-care. But as the saying goes, you can't pour from an empty cup – in order to show up fully for the people and things that matter most to us, we need to make sure we're taking care of ourselves first.

Self-care can take many different forms, depending on our individual needs and preferences. It might include things like getting enough sleep, eating nourishing foods, moving our bodies regularly, spending time in nature, or engaging in creative pursuits that bring us joy and fulfillment.

But self-care is not just about the big-picture practices that we engage in on a daily or weekly basis – it's also about the small, in-the-moment choices we make to prioritize our own well-being. That's where the power of aromatherapy and the Sensory Shift Method comes in – by incorporating simple, sensory self-care practices into our daily routines, we can create a sense of ritual and intention that helps us stay grounded and centered, even in the midst of stress.

For example, we might start our day with an energizing aromatherapy shower, using a blend of essential oils like grapefruit, eucalyptus, and ginger to awaken our senses and set a positive tone for the day ahead. Or, we might take a few minutes in the middle of a busy workday to apply a calming essential oil blend to our pulse points, close our eyes, and take a few deep breaths, creating a mini-moment of relaxation and reset.

By combining the power of scent, mindset, and self-care, the Sensory Shift Method offers a holistic and personalized approach to stress management that can be easily integrated into even the busiest of lifestyles. But how exactly do we put this method into practice? Let's explore the steps for crafting your own personal Sensory Shift ritual.

Crafting Your Personal Sensory Shift Ritual: Step-by-Step Guidance

One of the greatest strengths of the Sensory Shift Method is its adaptability – because it's based on the power of your own senses and personal preferences, it can be customized to fit your unique needs and lifestyle. But if you're new to aromatherapy or the Sensory Shift Method, the process of crafting your own personal ritual can feel a bit daunting.

That's why we've created a simple, step-by-step guide to help you get started. Here's how it works:

Step 1: Identify your stress triggers and symptoms. Before you can create a personalized Sensory Shift ritual, you need to have a clear understanding of what stress looks and feels like for you. Take some time to reflect on the situations, people, or experiences that tend to trigger feelings of stress, anxiety, or overwhelm for you. What are the physical, mental, and emotional symptoms that you experience when you're stressed? Do you feel tightness in your chest, a racing heart, or shallow breathing? Do you experience mental fog, difficulty concentrating, or negative self-talk? Do you feel irritable, tearful, or emotionally reactive? By getting clear on your personal stress triggers and symptoms, you can begin to identify the specific essential oils and self-care practices that will be most effective for you.

Step 2: Choose your essential oils. Once you have a clear understanding of your stress triggers and symptoms, it's time to choose the essential oils that will form the basis of your Sensory Shift ritual. As we explored in the previous chapter, different essential oils have different therapeutic properties and effects on the mind and body. Some oils, like lavender and bergamot, are known for their calming and relaxing effects, while others, like peppermint and rosemary, are more energizing and invigorating. Consider your personal preferences and sensitivities, as well as any specific health concerns or contraindications, when selecting your oils. You might choose a single oil that resonates with you, or create a custom blend that incorporates several different oils for a more complex and layered scent.

Step 3: Decide on your application method. There are many different ways to use essential oils for aromatherapy, from diffusing them in a room to applying them topically to the skin. Consider your personal preferences and lifestyle when deciding on your application method. If you spend a lot of time at a desk or in a small space, a diffuser might be a great option for creating a calming or uplifting atmosphere. If you're always on the go, a portable aromatherapy inhaler or rollerball might be more convenient for use throughout the day. If you enjoy the sensory experience of touch, an aromatherapy massage or bath might be more appealing. Experiment with different application methods to find what works best for you.

Step 4: Create your ritual. Once you've chosen your essential oils and application method, it's time to create your personal Sensory Shift ritual. This might be a simple, 30-second practice that you do every time you feel stressed, or a more elaborate, 10-minute self-care session that you incorporate into your daily routine. The key is to make your ritual feel intentional, meaningful, and enjoyable for you.

You might start by finding a quiet, comfortable space where you can sit or lie down without distractions. Take a few deep breaths, inhaling the scent of your chosen essential oils and allowing yourself to fully experience the sensations and emotions that arise. You might repeat a calming mantra or affirmation, visualize a peaceful scene, or simply focus on the rhythm of your breath. Allow yourself to be fully present in the moment, releasing any tension or stress and cultivating a sense of calm and balance.

Step 5: Integrate your ritual into your daily life. The real power of the Sensory Shift Method comes from consistent, daily practice. Look for opportunities to integrate your personal ritual into your existing routines and habits, whether it's first thing in the morning, during your lunch break, or before bed at night. Set reminders or cues for yourself to practice your ritual regularly, even when you're not feeling particularly stressed. Over time, this consistent practice can help to rewire your brain and nervous system, creating a more resilient and adaptable response to stress.

Cultivating Mindfulness and Gratitude: The Mental Shift

While the sensory experience of aromatherapy can be incredibly powerful for shifting our emotional state in the moment, the Sensory Shift Method is not just about quick fixes or temporary relief. It's also about cultivating a more positive, resilient, and grateful mindset that can help us navigate the challenges of life with greater ease and grace.

One of the key practices for cultivating this mindset is mindfulness, or the act of bringing our full attention and awareness to the present moment, without judgment or distraction. When we're stressed, our minds tend to race with worries about the future or regrets about the past, pulling us out of the present and creating a sense of disconnection and overwhelm.

By practicing mindfulness, we can learn to anchor ourselves in the present moment, observing our thoughts and emotions without getting caught up in them. This allows us to respond to stress with greater clarity, perspective, and intention, rather than simply reacting on autopilot.

Incorporating mindfulness into your Sensory Shift ritual can be as simple as taking a few deep breaths and noticing the sensations of the essential oils on your skin or in your nose. You might also try a brief body scan, systematically bringing your attention to each part of your body and releasing any tension or tightness you notice.

Another powerful practice for cultivating a positive mindset is gratitude, or the act of actively noticing and appreciating the good things in our lives. When we're stressed, it's easy to focus on all the things that are going wrong or the challenges we're facing, leading to a sense of scarcity and negativity.

By intentionally shifting our focus to the things we're grateful for, no matter how small, we can begin to cultivate a sense of abundance, joy, and perspective. This might be as simple as taking a moment each day to write down three things you're grateful for, or sharing your appreciation with others through kind words or acts of service.

Incorporating gratitude into your Sensory Shift ritual can be as simple as taking a moment to reflect on the things you're grateful for while inhaling your chosen essential oils. You might also try combining aromatherapy with other gratitude practices, like keeping a gratitude journal or sharing your appreciation with loved ones.

By combining the power of scent, mindfulness, and gratitude, the Sensory Shift Method offers a holistic approach to stress management that goes beyond just symptom relief. It's about cultivating a more positive, resilient, and empowered mindset that can help us thrive in the face of life's challenges.

Alright, let's make this a bit more down-to-earth. If you're looking to change how you deal with stress and want to feel more relaxed, clear-headed, and happy, why not give the Sensory Shift Method a whirl? You can create a little routine for yourself with the tips we've talked about. Try bringing a bit of mindfulness and thankfulness into your everyday routine and see if you notice a change in how you feel after a while.

Remember, stress is a natural and inevitable part of life – but it doesn't have to control or define us. By harnessing the power of our own senses, mindset, and self-care practices, we can learn to navigate stress with greater ease, resilience, and grace. The Sensory Shift Method is here to support you every step of the way.

Chapter 4

The 7-Day Reset: Your Journey to Transformed Stress Management

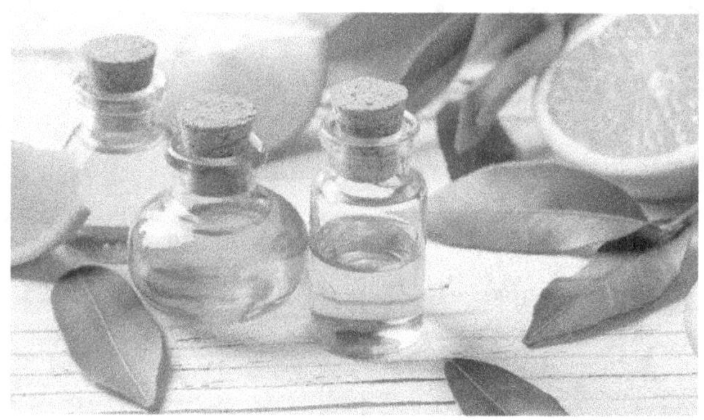

Are you ready to take your stress management to the next level? To not just survive the challenges of daily life, but to truly thrive in the face of them? If so, you're in the right place. Welcome to the 7-Day Reset: a transformative journey that will guide you through the process of integrating the Sensory Shift Method into your daily life, one day at a time.

Over the course of the next seven days, you'll be exploring a series of simple, yet powerful practices that combine the science of aromatherapy with the art of mindfulness and self-care. Each day will focus on a different aspect of stress management, from setting intentions and creating sacred space, to cultivating resilience and navigating challenges with grace.

But before we dive into the details of each day's practice, let's take a moment to set the stage for your journey. Because the truth is, transforming your relationship with stress isn't just about what you do – it's also about how you approach it.

Day 1: Setting Intentions and Creating a Sacred Space

The first step in any transformative journey is to get clear on your intentions. What do you hope to gain from this experience? What does a life of greater calm, balance, and resilience look like for you? Take some time to reflect on these questions, and to set a clear, positive intention for your 7-Day Reset.

Maybe your intention is to cultivate a greater sense of inner peace, even in the midst of chaos. Maybe it's to develop a more compassionate and nurturing relationship with yourself, one that prioritizes self-care and self-love. Maybe it's to build greater resilience and adaptability, so that you can navigate life's challenges with greater ease and grace.

Whatever your intention may be, take a moment to write it down, and to connect with the feelings and emotions that arise when you imagine yourself embodying that intention fully. Allow yourself to feel the excitement, the hope, and the possibility that comes with embarking on this journey.

Once you've set your intention, it's time to create a sacred space for your practice. This doesn't have to be a literal space (although it certainly can be) – it's more about creating a sense of intentionality and reverence around your self-care practice.

You might choose to create a physical altar or sanctuary in your home, complete with candles, crystals, and inspiring images or objects. Or you might simply set aside a quiet corner of your bedroom or office, where you can sit undisturbed for a few minutes each day.

The key is to create a space that feels sacred and special to you –

a space that invites you to slow down, to breathe deeply, and to connect with yourself on a deeper level. Take some time to cultivate this space, and to infuse it with your own personal touches and aesthetic.

As you begin your practice for the day, take a moment to light a candle, to set an intention, or to simply take a few deep breaths in your sacred space. Allow yourself to arrive fully in the present moment, and to open yourself up to the transformative power of the Sensory Shift Method.

Today's Practice:

- Set a clear, positive intention for your 7-Day Reset journey
- Create a sacred space for your daily practice, whether physical or symbolic
- Light a candle, set an intention, or take a few deep breaths to arrive fully in the present moment
- Use the Sensory Shift blend for Day 1: Grounding (vetiver, frankincense, and cedarwood)

Day 2-6: Building Momentum and Embracing the Shift

Over the course of the next five days, you'll be exploring a series of different Sensory Shift blends and practices, each designed to support a different aspect of stress management and resilience.

On Day 2, you'll be focusing on the theme of Clarity, using a blend of peppermint, rosemary, and lemon to cut through mental fog, boost focus and concentration, and inspire creative problem-solving. You might choose to incorporate this blend into a morning yoga or meditation practice, or to use it throughout the day to help you stay on task and motivated.

On Day 3, the theme is Balance, using a blend of lavender, bergamot, and ylang-ylang to promote a sense of calm, harmony, and emotional equilibrium. This is a great blend to use during times of transition or stress, when you need to find your center and maintain a sense of inner peace.

Day 4 focuses on the theme of Energy, using a blend of grapefruit, eucalyptus, and ginger to awaken your senses, boost your vitality, and help you power through even the most challenging of days. You might choose to incorporate this blend into a morning shower or workout routine, or to use it as a pick-me-up during an afternoon slump.

On Day 5, the theme is Resilience, using a blend of frankincense, sandalwood, and myrrh to cultivate a sense of inner strength, courage, and adaptability. This is a powerful blend to use during times of adversity or uncertainty, when you need to tap into your own deep reserves of resilience and grit.

Finally, on Day 6, the theme is Joy, using a blend of wild orange, jasmine, and vanilla to uplift your spirits, inspire positivity, and cultivate a sense of playfulness and lightheartedness. This is a wonderful blend to use when you need a boost of optimism or inspiration, or simply want to infuse more joy and laughter into your day.

Throughout these five days, you'll be incorporating a variety of different self-care practices and rituals into your daily routine, from aromatherapy showers and baths to mindfulness meditations and gratitude journaling. You'll also be exploring different ways to use your Sensory Shift blends, from diffusing them in your home or office to applying them topically to your pulse points or chakras.

The key is to approach each day's practice with a sense of curiosity, openness, and self-compassion. Remember, this is not about perfection or achieving some kind of magical transformation overnight. It's about showing up for yourself, day after day, and taking small, consistent steps towards greater resilience, balance, and joy.

Every day you practice, pay attention to how you're feeling—your mood, how much pep you've got, or just how good you're feeling in general. Give yourself a pat on the back for the wins, even the tiny ones, and don't be too hard on yourself if things get tough.

Remember, transformation is not a linear process – it's a journey of ups and downs, twists and turns. Trust that each step is taking you closer to your intention, and that the Sensory Shift Method is there to support you every step of the way.

Day 7: Reflecting, Celebrating, and Planning for Lasting Change

Congratulations! You've made it to the final day of your 7-Day Reset. Take a moment to acknowledge and celebrate all the hard work, dedication, and self-care you've put in over the past week. Whether you've experienced profound shifts or subtle changes, every step you've taken has been a step towards greater resilience, balance, and joy.

Today is a day for reflection, integration, and planning for the future. Take some time to look back on your journey, and to assess what worked well for you and what didn't. What practices or rituals felt most nourishing and supportive? What challenges or obstacles did you face, and how did you navigate them?

Consider journaling about your experiences, or sharing your reflections with a trusted friend or family member. Allow yourself to fully acknowledge and celebrate your successes, and to learn from any setbacks or challenges you faced.

Looking forward to what's coming, think about making the Sensory Shift Method a regular part of your routine. What little things can you do every day to make sure you're taking care of yourself and keeping stress at bay, no matter what life throws at you?

Maybe it's committing to a daily aromatherapy ritual, or incorporating mindfulness practices into your morning routine. Maybe it's setting boundaries around your time and energy, or creating a regular self-care date with yourself. Maybe it's finding a community of like-minded individuals who can support and encourage you on your journey.

Whatever your plan may be, remember that lasting change is not about perfection or overnight transformation – it's about consistency, self-compassion, and a willingness to show up for yourself, day after day.

You've made it through the 7-Day Reset! Take a little time to think back on why you started and what you wanted to achieve. Now's the perfect chance to think about what's next. Get excited about the new doors that are opening for you, the balance you're bringing into your life, and all the happiness that's waiting for you. Keep that feeling close as you move forward.

And remember, the Sensory Shift Method is always here to support you, whenever you need it. Whether you're facing a particularly stressful day or simply need a moment of self-care and reflection, you now have a powerful tool at your fingertips – one that can help you navigate life's challenges with greater ease, grace, and resilience.

So here's to you, my friend – to your courage, your dedication, and your unwavering commitment to your own well-being. May the Sensory Shift Method be a constant companion on your journey, and may you always remember the incredible power and potential that lies within you.

Today's Practice:

- Reflect on your 7-Day Reset journey, acknowledging successes and learning from challenges
- Consider how you can integrate the Sensory Shift Method into your daily life moving forward
- Set a new intention for the journey ahead, and recommit to your own well-being and resilience
- Use the Sensory Shift blend for Day 7: Gratitude (frankincense, myrrh, and orange)
- Celebrate your incredible accomplishment, and trust in the journey ahead

I just wanted to share a couple of last thoughts and a bit of a pep talk as we wrap up our 7-Day Reset. It's been quite the journey, hasn't it? I hope you're feeling as refreshed and motivated as I am.

Let's take everything we've learned and make the most of it. Here's to new beginnings and the exciting path ahead!

First, remember that stress is a natural and inevitable part of life – but it doesn't have to control or define you. With the tools and practices of the Sensory Shift Method, you now have the power to navigate stress with greater ease, resilience, and grace. Trust in your own strength and capacity, and know that you are never alone on this journey.

Second, be patient and compassionate with yourself as you continue to integrate these practices into your daily life. Transformation is not a destination, but a lifelong journey of growth, learning, and self-discovery. Embrace the ebbs and flows, the ups and downs, and trust that each step is taking you closer to your highest self.

And finally, remember that self-care is not selfish – it's essential. By prioritizing your own well-being and resilience, you are not only caring for yourself, but also creating a ripple effect of positive change in the world around you. When you show up as your best self, you inspire others to do the same – and together, we can create a world of greater compassion, connection, and joy.

So thank you, my friend, for showing up for yourself and for this journey. Thank you for your courage, your commitment, and your willingness to embrace a new way of being. And thank you for being a part of this incredible community of resilient, compassionate, and inspiring individuals.

I hope that the 7-Day Reset has been a transformative and empowering experience for you, and that the Sensory Shift Method will continue to be a valuable tool and companion on your journey ahead. Remember, I am always here to support and encourage you, every step of the way.

Chapter 5

Essential Oils for Every Occasion: Targeted Blends for Specific Stressors

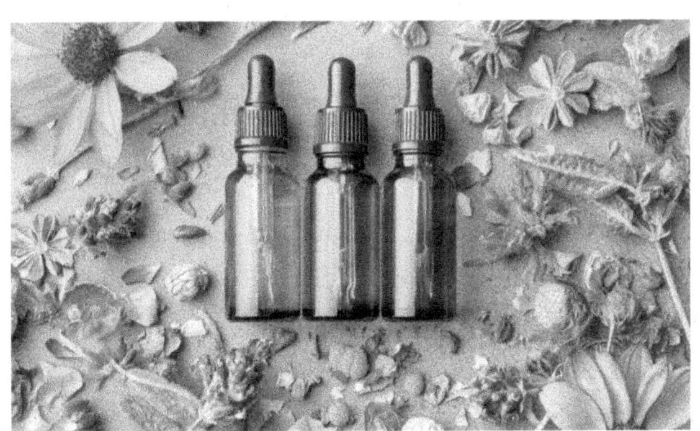

In the previous chapters, we've explored the powerful role that essential oils and aromatherapy can play in managing stress, cultivating resilience, and promoting overall well-being. From the science behind the olfactory system to the art of crafting a personalized Sensory Shift ritual, we've laid the foundation for a holistic and effective approach to stress management.

But what about those specific stressors and challenges that arise in our daily lives? The ones that can throw us off balance, drain our energy, and leave us feeling overwhelmed and depleted? Whether it's a looming deadline at work, a difficult conversation with a loved one, or the constant juggle of multiple responsibilities, we all face unique stressors that require targeted support and care.

That's where the power of specific essential oil blends comes in. By combining the right oils in the right proportions, we can create targeted blends that address the specific physical, emotional, and mental symptoms of different stressors, providing us with a powerful tool for navigating life's challenges with greater ease and resilience.

In this chapter, we'll be exploring some of the most common stressors that high-achieving women face, and the specific essential oil blends that can help alleviate their symptoms and promote greater balance and well-being. From work stress and relationship challenges to caregiver fatigue and more, we'll be diving deep into the world of targeted aromatherapy, empowering you with the knowledge and tools you need to thrive in the face of any stressor.

Work Stress: Blends for Focus, Clarity, and Confidence

Let's face it: work stress is a reality for most of us, especially in today's fast-paced, high-pressure world. Whether you're an entrepreneur, a corporate executive, or anything in between, the demands of work can take a toll on our mental, emotional, and physical well-being, leaving us feeling drained, anxious, and overwhelmed.

But with the right essential oil blends, we can help mitigate the effects of work stress, promoting greater focus, clarity, and confidence in the face of even the toughest challenges. Here are a few of our favorite blends for work stress:

1. "Laser Focus" Blend: Combine 3 drops of peppermint, 2 drops of rosemary, and 1 drop of lemon to create a blend that promotes mental clarity, focus, and concentration. This blend is perfect for those times when you need to

power through a challenging project or task, providing a
natural boost of energy and alertness.

2. "Confident Leadership" Blend: Combine 3 drops of
   bergamot, 2 drops of frankincense, and 1 drop of ylang-
   ylang to create a blend that promotes confidence, self-
   assurance, and inner strength. This blend is great for
   those moments when you need to step into your power as
   a leader, whether you're giving a presentation, leading a
   team, or advocating for yourself and your ideas.

3. "Stress Relief" Blend: Combine 3 drops of lavender, 2
   drops of clary sage, and 1 drop of Roman chamomile to
   create a blend that promotes relaxation, calm, and
   emotional balance. This blend is perfect for those times
   when work stress is taking a toll on your mental and
   emotional well-being, helping you release tension and
   find a sense of inner peace.

To use these blends, simply add the appropriate number of drops
to your diffuser, or mix with a carrier oil and apply topically to your
pulse points or temples. Take a few deep breaths, allowing the aroma
to fill your senses and promote a sense of calm, focus, and confidence.

Relationship Stress: Blends for Emotional Balance and Harmony

Our relationships with others – whether romantic, familial, or
platonic – are often a source of great joy and fulfillment in our lives.
But they can also be a source of significant stress and emotional
turmoil, particularly when conflicts arise or communication breaks
down.

During times of relationship stress, it's essential to prioritize our
own emotional well-being and cultivate a sense of inner balance and
harmony. And with the right essential oil blends, we can support

ourselves in navigating even the most challenging relational dynamics with greater ease and grace.

Here are a few of our favorite blends for relationship stress:

1. "Emotional Balance" Blend: Combine 3 drops of geranium, 2 drops of bergamot, and 1 drop of rose to create a blend that promotes emotional balance, stability, and inner peace. This blend is particularly useful during times of high stress or conflict, helping you stay centered and grounded in the face of difficult emotions.

2. "Heart Healing" Blend: Combine 3 drops of ylang-ylang, 2 drops of lavender, and 1 drop of neroli to create a blend that promotes emotional healing, forgiveness, and compassion. This blend is great for those times when you're working through a difficult relational challenge, helping you cultivate a sense of openness, understanding, and empathy.

3. "Boundary Setting" Blend: Combine 3 drops of grapefruit, 2 drops of lemongrass, and 1 drop of peppermint to create a blend that promotes clarity, assertiveness, and healthy boundaries. This blend is particularly useful when you need to have a difficult conversation or set clear limits in a relationship, helping you communicate your needs and desires with confidence and grace.

As with the work stress blends, simply add the appropriate number of drops to your diffuser or mix with a carrier oil for topical application. Take a few moments to breathe deeply and connect with your inner sense of calm, balance, and strength.

Caregiver Stress: Blends for Resilience and Self-Compassion

For many women, the role of caregiver – whether for children, aging parents, or other loved ones – is a deeply meaningful and rewarding one. But it can also be incredibly stressful, demanding, and emotionally draining, particularly when paired with the many other responsibilities and roles we juggle on a daily basis.

Taking care of others means we've got to take care of ourselves too. It's like making sure our own 'tank' is full so we can be there for our loved ones in the best way possible. Using the right mix of essential oils can really help us build the emotional strength and clearheadedness we need to handle the ups and downs of looking after someone. It's all about making the journey a little smoother for ourselves.

Here are a few of our favorite blends for caregiver stress:

1. "Resilience" Blend: Combine 3 drops of frankincense, 2 drops of sandalwood, and 1 drop of helichrysum to create a blend that promotes emotional resilience, inner strength, and the ability to bounce back from stress and adversity. This blend is perfect for those times when you're feeling overwhelmed or depleted by the demands of caregiving, helping you tap into your own deep reserves of strength and resilience.
2. "Self-Compassion" Blend: Combine 3 drops of rose, 2 drops of neroli, and 1 drop of lavender to create a blend that promotes self-love, self-acceptance, and self-compassion. This blend is great for those moments when you're feeling critical of yourself or your caregiving abilities, helping you cultivate a sense of kindness and understanding towards yourself.
3. "Renewal" Blend: Combine 3 drops of lemon, 2 drops of peppermint, and 1 drop of rosemary to create a blend

that promotes mental clarity, energy, and a sense of renewal. This blend is particularly useful when you're feeling mentally or physically fatigued from the demands of caregiving, helping you refresh and recharge your batteries.

Use these blends in your diffuser or mixed with a carrier oil for topical application, taking a few moments to breathe deeply and connect with your inner sense of strength, compassion, and resilience.

Other Stressors and Blends

Of course, work stress, relationship stress, and caregiver stress are just a few examples of the many stressors that high-achieving women face on a daily basis. From financial stress and health concerns to environmental stressors and more, the list of potential stressors is virtually endless.

But no matter what specific stressor you may be facing, there is likely an essential oil blend that can help support you in navigating it with greater ease and resilience. Here are a few more examples of targeted blends for specific stressors:

1. Financial Stress Blend: Combine 3 drops of grapefruit, 2 drops of frankincense, and 1 drop of bergamot to create a blend that promotes abundance, clarity, and trust in the face of financial stress and uncertainty.
2. Health Concern Blend: Combine 3 drops of lavender, 2 drops of frankincense, and 1 drop of tea tree to create a blend that promotes relaxation, immune support, and emotional balance during times of health-related stress and worry.
3. Environmental Stress Blend: Combine 3 drops of lemon, 2 drops of eucalyptus, and 1 drop of tea tree to create a

blend that promotes mental clarity, respiratory support, and a sense of freshness and renewal in the face of environmental stressors like pollution or allergens.

The key is to get creative and experiment with different blends and combinations that resonate with your specific needs and preferences. Trust your intuition and pay attention to how different oils and blends make you feel, both physically and emotionally.

Remember that essential oils can be really helpful for dealing with stress and making you feel better, but they're not a replacement for seeing a doctor or a therapist if you're dealing with serious or long-lasting stress, anxiety, or any other mental health issues. If that's what you're going through, it's important to get help from a professional.

Chapter 6

Integrating Aromatherapy into Your Lifestyle: Beyond the 7-Day Reset

Congratulations on completing the 7-Day Reset! By now, you've experienced firsthand the transformative power of essential oils and the Sensory Shift Method in managing stress, cultivating resilience, and promoting overall well-being. You've learned how to craft personalized blends, create sacred self-care rituals, and navigate specific stressors with the help of targeted aromatherapy solutions.

But the journey doesn't end here. In fact, the real magic happens when we integrate these practices into our daily lives, creating sustainable habits and rituals that support us in showing up as our best selves, no matter what challenges come our way.

In this chapter, we'll explore practical strategies for weaving aromatherapy and the Sensory Shift Method into your lifestyle, beyond the structure of the 7-Day Reset. From morning routines and nighttime rituals to workplace wellness and travel essentials, we'll cover a wide range of ways to make aromatherapy a seamless part of your daily life.

Aromatherapy for Better Sleep: Blends and Rituals for Restful Nights

One of the most powerful ways to integrate aromatherapy into your lifestyle is to harness its potential for promoting deep, restful sleep. In today's fast-paced world, many of us struggle with sleep issues, from difficulty falling asleep to frequent waking or restless nights. Over time, these disruptions can take a toll on our physical, mental, and emotional well-being, contributing to feelings of stress, anxiety, and burnout.

But with the right essential oil blends and bedtime rituals, we can signal to our bodies and minds that it's time to unwind, relax, and drift off into peaceful slumber. Here are a few of our favorite blends and rituals for promoting better sleep:

1. "Lavender Lullaby" Blend: Combine 3 drops of lavender, 2 drops of bergamot, and 1 drop of ylang-ylang to create a soothing and calming blend that promotes relaxation and restful sleep. Add this blend to your diffuser or mix with a carrier oil for a gentle bedtime massage.
2. "Sweet Dreams" Pillow Spray: In a small spray bottle, combine 10 drops of lavender, 5 drops of chamomile, and 5 drops of marjoram with 2 ounces of distilled water. Shake well and spritz lightly on your pillow and sheets before bedtime for a calming and comforting aroma.
3. Bedtime Foot Massage Ritual: In a small bowl, mix 2 drops of lavender, 2 drops of frankincense, and 1 drop of vetiver with 1 tablespoon of carrier oil (such as coconut or jojoba). Gently massage this blend into your feet and toes, taking deep breaths and allowing the aroma to fill your senses. This grounding and relaxing ritual is perfect for signaling to your body that it's time to rest and unwind.

In addition to these blends and rituals, it's important to create a sleep-friendly environment that supports your body's natural rhythms and promotes feelings of calm and tranquility. This might include investing in comfortable bedding, keeping your bedroom cool and dark, and minimizing exposure to electronic devices and stimulating activities before bedtime.

Aromatherapy for Energizing Mornings: Blends and Rituals for a Positive Start

Just as aromatherapy can help us unwind and relax at the end of the day, it can also be a powerful tool for energizing and uplifting us in the morning. Starting our day with intentional self-care rituals and invigorating essential oil blends can help set a positive tone for the day ahead, boosting our mood, focus, and motivation.

Here are a few of our favorite blends and rituals for energizing mornings:

1. "Rise and Shine" Blend: Combine 3 drops of peppermint, 2 drops of lemon, and 1 drop of rosemary to create an invigorating and uplifting blend that promotes mental clarity and energy. Add this blend to your diffuser or mix with a carrier oil for an energizing morning massage.
2. "Sunny Citrus" Body Scrub: In a small bowl, mix 1/2 cup of sugar, 1/4 cup of coconut oil, 5 drops of sweet orange, and 5 drops of grapefruit. Use this refreshing and exfoliating scrub in the shower for a burst of energizing citrus aroma and smooth, radiant skin.
3. Morning Mindfulness Ritual: Before starting your day, take a few moments to sit in a quiet space and engage in a simple mindfulness practice. Hold a bottle of your favorite energizing essential oil (such as peppermint, lemon, or eucalyptus) and take a few deep breaths,

allowing the aroma to fill your senses. As you breathe, set a positive intention for the day ahead, visualizing yourself moving through your tasks and interactions with ease, grace, and joy.

Incorporating these energizing blends and rituals into your morning routine can help you start your day with a sense of purpose, clarity, and vitality, setting the stage for a more productive and fulfilling day ahead.

Aromatherapy for Mindful Moments: Blends and Rituals for Presence and Calm

In the midst of our busy, fast-paced lives, it can be all too easy to get caught up in the whirlwind of our thoughts, worries, and to-do lists. We may find ourselves constantly rushing from one task to the next, feeling disconnected from our bodies, our emotions, and the present moment.

This is where the power of mindfulness comes in. By taking intentional pauses throughout our day to tune in to our senses, our breath, and our surroundings, we can cultivate a greater sense of presence, calm, and inner peace. And when we combine mindfulness practices with the transformative power of aromatherapy, we create a potent tool for navigating stress and cultivating resilience.

Here are a few of our favorite blends and rituals for mindful moments:

1. "Grounding" Blend: Combine 3 drops of frankincense, 2 drops of cedarwood, and 1 drop of vetiver to create a grounding and centering blend that promotes feelings of calm, stability, and inner peace. Use this blend in your diffuser or mix with a carrier oil for a soothing massage.
2. "Breath of Fresh Air" Mist: In a small spray bottle, combine 10 drops of eucalyptus, 5 drops of peppermint,

and 5 drops of lemon with 2 ounces of distilled water. Shake well and spritz around your face and neck for a refreshing and invigorating aroma that promotes mental clarity and deep breathing.

3. Mindful Walking Ritual: Take a short break from your workday to step outside and engage in a mindful walking practice. As you walk, pay attention to the sensations of your feet hitting the ground, the rhythm of your breath, and the sights, sounds, and smells around you. Carry a small bottle of your favorite grounding or uplifting essential oil blend and take a few deep breaths, allowing the aroma to anchor you in the present moment.

By incorporating these mindful moments and aromatherapy practices into your daily routine, you create opportunities to pause, breathe, and reconnect with yourself and your surroundings. Over time, these small acts of presence and self-care can add up to a greater sense of overall well-being, resilience, and joy.

Aromatherapy in the Workplace: Blends and Strategies for Focus and Stress Relief

For many of us, the workplace can be a significant source of stress, with endless deadlines, meetings, and demands competing for our time and energy. But what if we could harness the power of aromatherapy to create a more positive, productive, and stress-free work environment?

By incorporating essential oil blends and mindful practices into our workday, we can promote greater focus, creativity, and resilience, even in the face of challenging projects or difficult conversations. Here are a few strategies and blends to try:

1. "Focus and Clarity" Blend: Combine 3 drops of peppermint, 2 drops of lemon, and 1 drop of basil to

create a blend that promotes mental clarity, focus, and concentration. Add this blend to a personal diffuser or inhale directly from the bottle before tackling a challenging task or project.

2. "Stress Relief" Roller Blend: In a 10ml roller bottle, combine 10 drops of lavender, 5 drops of bergamot, and 5 drops of frankincense with a carrier oil (such as fractionated coconut oil). Roll this blend onto your pulse points (wrists, neck, temples) throughout the day for a quick and easy stress relief boost.

3. Mindful Meeting Practice: Before entering a potentially stressful meeting or conversation, take a few moments to center yourself with a simple mindfulness practice. Close your eyes, take a few deep breaths, and visualize yourself moving through the interaction with calm, clarity, and compassion. You might also apply a grounding or uplifting essential oil blend to your pulse points for an added layer of aromatic support.

In addition to these individual practices, consider advocating for the use of aromatherapy in your workplace as a whole. This might include adding essential oil diffusers to common areas, creating a "calm room" with soothing scents and relaxing music, or offering aromatherapy workshops or resources to your colleagues.

By bringing the power of aromatherapy into the workplace, we create a more supportive, nurturing, and stress-free environment for ourselves and our colleagues, leading to greater productivity, creativity, and overall job satisfaction.

Aromatherapy on the Go: Travel Essentials and Blends for Balance and Comfort

Whether for work or pleasure, travel can be an exciting and enriching experience – but it can also be a significant source of stress and discomfort. From long flights and jet lag to unfamiliar environments and disrupted routines, the challenges of travel can take a toll on our physical, mental, and emotional well-being.

But with the right aromatherapy essentials and travel-friendly blends, we can create a sense of comfort, balance, and home-away-from-home wherever our journeys may take us. Here are a few must-have items and blends for your aromatherapy travel kit:

1. "Immune Support" Roll-On Blend: In a 10ml roller bottle, combine 10 drops of tea tree, 5 drops of lemon, and 5 drops of eucalyptus with a carrier oil. Apply this protective and refreshing blend to your pulse points and bottoms of your feet before and during travel to support your immune system and promote respiratory health.
2. "Jet Lag Relief" Inhaler Blend: In a blank aromatherapy inhaler, add 10 drops of peppermint, 8 drops of rosemary, and 6 drops of grapefruit. Inhale deeply from this energizing and clarifying blend to help reset your internal clock and combat feelings of jet lag and fatigue.
3. Portable Diffuser and "Relaxation" Blend: Invest in a small, USB-powered diffuser that can easily fit in your carry-on luggage. Fill with water and add 2-3 drops of a calming blend, such as 3 drops of lavender, 2 drops of bergamot, and 1 drop of ylang-ylang, to create a soothing and relaxing atmosphere in your hotel room or vacation rental.

Before you set off on your travels, why not start a little tradition for yourself? It's like your personal send-off ritual. You could think about what you hope to get out of the trip, maybe take a couple of deep breaths with a scent that makes you feel steady or cheerful, or even spend a few minutes just being present or stretching out with some yoga. It's a nice way to get your head and heart in the right place before you take off.

By making aromatherapy a part of your travel routine, you create a sense of continuity and self-care that can help you feel more grounded, balanced, and at ease, no matter where your adventures may take you.

Chapter 7

The Art of Blending: Creating Your Own Signature Scents

Throughout this book, we've explored the incredible power of essential oils and aromatherapy to transform our lives, one breath at a time. From the science of scent and the emotional impact of aroma to the practical applications of targeted blends and lifestyle rituals, we've covered a wide range of topics and techniques designed to help you harness the magic of essential oils for greater well-being, resilience, and joy.

But now, it's time to take your aromatherapy practice to the next level by diving into the art of blending – the creative process of combining individual essential oils to create your own unique and personalized scents. Blending is where the true magic of aromatherapy lies, as it allows you to tap into your own intuition, creativity, and sensory preferences to craft scents that are perfectly tailored to your needs and desires.

In this chapter, we'll explore the fundamental principles and techniques of blending, as well as provide you with a step-by-step guide to creating your own signature scents. Whether you're a beginner or an experienced aromatherapy enthusiast, this chapter will give you the tools and inspiration you need to unleash your inner perfumer and create scents that are truly one-of-a-kind.

Understanding Essential Oil Notes and Families

The first step in mastering the art of blending is to understand the basic building blocks of scent – essential oil notes and families. Just like in music, where individual notes come together to create chords and melodies, essential oils can be classified into different "notes" based on their aromatic characteristics and how quickly they evaporate.

There are three main categories of essential oil notes:

1. Top Notes: These are the lightest and most volatile oils, which means they are the first to evaporate and the first scents you smell in a blend. Top notes are often described as fresh, bright, and uplifting, and they tend to have a strong initial impact but fade quickly. Examples of top note oils include citrus oils like lemon, lime, and bergamot, as well as light florals like lavender and eucalyptus.
2. Middle Notes: Also known as "heart notes," these oils are the foundation of a blend and make up the majority of the scent. They are often described as warm, soft, and well-rounded, and they tend to have a longer-lasting aroma that emerges after the top notes have faded. Examples of middle note oils include floral oils like rose, geranium, and ylang-ylang, as well as herbaceous oils like rosemary, lavender, and clary sage.
3. Base Notes: These are the heaviest and least volatile oils, which means they are the last to evaporate and the scents that linger the longest. Base notes are often described as deep, rich, and grounding, and they help to anchor and stabilize a blend. Examples of base note oils include

woody oils like cedarwood, sandalwood, and patchouli, as well as resinous oils like frankincense and myrrh.

In addition to notes, essential oils can also be grouped into different "families" based on their aromatic qualities and the types of plants they come from. The main essential oil families include:

1. Citrus: Bright, fresh, and uplifting scents like lemon, orange, grapefruit, and bergamot.
2. Floral: Soft, sweet, and romantic scents like rose, jasmine, ylang-ylang, and geranium.
3. Herbaceous: Fresh, green, and earthy scents like lavender, rosemary, peppermint, and basil.
4. Woody: Deep, warm, and grounding scents like cedarwood, sandalwood, pine, and cypress.
5. Spicy: Warm, energizing, and exotic scents like cinnamon, ginger, clove, and black pepper.
6. Resinous: Rich, complex, and spiritual scents like frankincense, myrrh, and benzoin.

Understanding the different notes and families of essential oils is key to creating well-balanced and harmonious blends. A good general rule of thumb is to include oils from each note category (top, middle, and base) in your blends, as well as to combine oils from complementary families (such as citrus and floral, or woody and spicy).

However, it's important to remember that blending is as much an art as it is a science, and there are no hard and fast rules. The most important thing is to trust your nose and your intuition, and to have fun experimenting with different combinations and ratios until you find a scent that feels just right to you.

The Basics of Blending: Ratios, Equipment, and Safety

Now that you have a basic understanding of essential oil notes and families, it's time to dive into the practical aspects of blending. Before you begin, it's important to gather the right equipment and materials, as well as to familiarize yourself with some basic blending ratios and safety guidelines.

Here's what you'll need to get started:

- Essential oils of your choice
- Carrier oils (such as fractionated coconut oil, jojoba oil, or sweet almond oil)
- Glass bottles or jars for storing your blends
- droppers or pipettes for measuring and mixing oils
- Labels and a pen for labeling your blends
- A notebook or journal for keeping track of your recipes and observations

When it comes to blending ratios, a good starting point is to use a 2:1:1 ratio of top, middle, and base note oils. For example, in a 10ml blend, you might use 4 drops of a top note oil, 2 drops of a middle note oil, and 2 drops of a base note oil.

However, this is just a general guideline, and you can adjust the ratios to suit your personal preferences and the specific oils you're working with. Some oils, like patchouli or ylang-ylang, have a stronger aroma and may require fewer drops, while others, like lavender or lemon, are more subtle and may require more.

Experimenting with different ratios and combinations is a lot like being a kitchen wizard, but even wizards need a good memory aid. So, jot down your recipes and any notes about how they turned out in a blending journal. This way, you can easily remember which concoctions were a hit and which ones flopped. Plus, when you stumble upon a blend you absolutely love, you'll have the recipe handy to whip it up again.

When it comes to safety, there are a few key guidelines to keep in mind when blending essential oils:

- Always dilute your essential oils in a carrier oil before applying them to your skin. A good general ratio is 2-3 drops of essential oil per teaspoon of carrier oil.
- Avoid using essential oils that are known to be skin irritants or sensitizers, such as cinnamon, clove, or thyme, in your blends.
- Be cautious when using essential oils around children, pregnant women, or people with sensitive skin or allergies. Always do a patch test before using a new blend, and consult with a qualified aromatherapist or healthcare provider if you have any concerns.
- Store your essential oils and blends in a cool, dark place away from direct sunlight and heat, as these can degrade the quality and potency of the oils over time.

By following these basic safety guidelines and using high-quality, pure essential oils, you can ensure that your blending practice is both enjoyable and effective.

Signature Scent Workshop: Step-by-Step Blending Guide

Now that you have your equipment and materials ready and understand the basics of blending ratios and safety, it's time to dive into the fun part – creating your own signature scent!

Here's a step-by-step guide to help you get started:

Step 1: Set an intention. Before you begin blending, take a moment to connect with your intuition and set an intention for your signature scent. What do you want this scent to represent or evoke?

How do you want to feel when you wear it? Write down your intention in your blending journal.

Step 2: Choose your oils. Based on your intention and your personal scent preferences, choose a selection of essential oils from different notes and families that you feel drawn to. Don't be afraid to mix and match oils from different categories – sometimes the most unexpected combinations can be the most beautiful!

Step 3: Prep your materials. Gather your chosen oils, carrier oil, blending equipment, and journal. Make sure your workspace is clean and well-ventilated.

Step 4: Start with your base note. In a clean glass bottle or jar, add 2-3 drops of your chosen base note oil. This will be the foundation of your blend and the scent that lingers the longest.

Step 5: Add your middle note. Next, add 4-5 drops of your chosen middle note oil to the blend. This will be the "heart" of your scent and the aroma that emerges after the top notes have faded.

Step 6: Finish with your top note. Finally, add 6-7 drops of your chosen top note oil to the blend. This will be the first scent you smell when you apply the blend and will give your signature scent its initial burst of aroma.

Step 7: Mix and adjust. Gently swirl or stir your blend to mix the oils together. Take a deep breath and inhale the aroma. How does it smell? Is it well-balanced, or does one note overpower the others? If needed, adjust the ratios of your oils until you achieve a scent that feels harmonious and pleasing to you.

Step 8: Dilute and test. Once you're happy with your blend, add enough carrier oil to dilute it to a safe concentration (usually 2-3% for body oils or perfumes). Label your blend with the name, date, and ingredients, and do a patch test on a small area of skin to make sure you don't have any adverse reactions.

Step 9: Refine and reflect. As you wear your signature scent over the next few days, take note of how it evolves and how it makes you feel. Do you find yourself reaching for it often, or does it feel like something is missing? Don't be afraid to tweak your recipe or start fresh with a new blend – the beauty of blending is that it's a constantly evolving and creative process!

Creating your own signature scent is all about enjoying the process. Trust your gut and let your imagination run wild. The more you play around with different blends, the more you'll find a style that's truly you. Just give it time, and before you know it, you'll have a fragrance that's a perfect expression of who you are.

Blending for Mood and Intention: Recipes and Ideas

Mixing essential oils isn't just about making a unique fragrance that's all your own. It's also a great tool for looking after your emotional health and bringing to life certain goals or wishes you have. When you pick out oils that have just the right smell and vibe for what you're after, you can whip up a blend that does wonders for your mood. Whether you're looking to feel more down-to-earth, get your head in the game, spark some creativity, or give yourself a boost of energy, there's a combination that can help you out right when you need it.

Here are a few ideas and recipes to get you started:

1. Grounding Blend: Combine 3 drops of vetiver, 2 drops of cedarwood, and 1 drop of frankincense for a blend that promotes feelings of stability, security, and inner peace. This blend is great for when you're feeling scattered or overwhelmed and need to reconnect with your center.
2. Focus Blend: Combine 3 drops of rosemary, 2 drops of peppermint, and 1 drop of lemon for a blend that promotes mental clarity, concentration, and memory. This blend is perfect for when you need to tackle a challenging project or study for an exam.
3. Inspiration Blend: Combine 3 drops of bergamot, 2 drops of ylang-ylang, and 1 drop of frankincense for a blend

that promotes creativity, intuition, and spiritual connection. This blend is great for when you're feeling stuck or uninspired and need a burst of fresh energy and ideas.

4. Energizing Blend: Combine 3 drops of grapefruit, 2 drops of peppermint, and 1 drop of rosemary for a blend that promotes vitality, enthusiasm, and physical energy. This blend is perfect for when you need a natural pick-me-up or a boost of motivation to tackle your day.

Absolutely, there's no limit to the creative mixes you can come up with! Play around with various scents and amounts, and take note of the vibes each one brings out in you. It could be fun to make a little ceremony out of using your blends too. Maybe think of a positive thought or a goal for the day as you put them on.

The most important thing is to approach blending with a sense of curiosity, playfulness, and self-discovery. Trust that your intuition will guide you to the perfect oils and combinations for your unique needs and desires, and have fun exploring the endless possibilities of scent and aroma.

Chapter 8

Empowered Self-Care: Embracing Your Inner Strength and Resilience

We're almost at the end of our exploration into essential oils and aromatherapy. I'd like to pause for a second and think about the amazing things we can do with just our sense of smell. This book has taken us through how scents can change the way we feel and think, and how they can even touch our souls. We've learned about how our noses work and the craft of mixing scents together.

But at the heart of this journey is a deeper message – one of self-care, self-love, and self-empowerment. Because the truth is, no matter how many blends we create or rituals we practice, true healing and transformation can only come from within. It's up to us to cultivate the inner strength, resilience, and wisdom that will guide us through life's challenges and help us thrive, no matter what comes our way.

In this final chapter, we'll explore what it means to embrace a truly empowered approach to self-care – one that goes beyond just the occasional bubble bath or spa day (though those are wonderful too!) and instead becomes a daily practice of nurturing our minds, bodies, and spirits from the inside out. We'll look at some of the key principles and practices of empowered self-care, as well as how to integrate aromatherapy and the Sensory Shift Method into a holistic, sustainable self-care routine.

So let's dive in and discover how we can unlock the full potential of our inner strength and resilience, one breath (and one drop of essential oil) at a time.

Redefining Self-Care: From Luxury to Necessity

For too long, self-care has been seen as a luxury – something that we might indulge in occasionally, if we have the time or money, but not something that we prioritize on a daily basis. We live in a culture that glorifies busyness and productivity, often at the expense of our own well-being and happiness. We're taught to put others' needs before our own, to push through the pain and exhaustion, and to feel guilty or selfish for taking time to rest and recharge.

But the truth is, self-care is not a luxury – it's a necessity. It's the foundation upon which all other aspects of our lives are built, from our physical health and mental well-being to our relationships, careers, and creative pursuits. When we neglect our own needs and desires, we become depleted, disconnected, and unable to show up fully in the world.

So what does it mean to redefine self-care as a necessity? It means making a conscious, intentional choice to prioritize our own well-being, even (and especially) when life gets busy or stressful. It means creating non-negotiable time and space in our schedules for activities that nourish and replenish us, whether that's a daily meditation prac-tice, a weekly yoga class, or a monthly massage.

It also means shifting our mindset around self-care from one of indulgence or selfishness to one of self-love and self-respect. When we truly value ourselves and our own well-being, taking care of ourselves becomes a natural expression of that love and respect. We start to see self-care not as something we "should" do, but as some-thing we want to do – a gift that we give ourselves each and every day.

Changing the way we think isn't something that happens quickly. It's a process that requires us to be patient, to keep at it, and to face up to the negative beliefs and habits that might have trapped us in a pattern of not looking after ourselves or even working against our own interests. But if we stick with it and really commit to making self-care an essential part of every day, we'll start to see amazing changes in how we feel and live.

The Ripple Effect: How Your Self-Care Practices Impact Others

One of the most powerful things about embracing empowered self-care is the ripple effect it can have on the world around us. When we take care of ourselves and show up as our best, most authentic selves, we naturally inspire others to do the same. We become a living example of what it means to prioritize self-love and self-respect, and we create a positive ripple of change that extends far beyond ourselves.

Think about it: how many times have you been inspired by someone who exudes a sense of inner peace, joy, and resilience, even in the face of life's challenges? How many times have you felt uplifted or energized simply by being in the presence of someone who radiates self-love and self-care?

When we commit to our own self-care practices, we become that person for others. We create a ripple effect of positive change that touches everyone we interact with, from our family and friends to our colleagues and community. We become a living example of what it means to thrive, not just survive, and we inspire others to do the same.

This is especially true for those of us in leadership or caregiver roles, whether that's as a parent, a manager, a teacher, or a healer. When we prioritize our own self-care and well-being, we become better equipped to show up fully and authentically for those we serve. We have more energy, patience, and compassion to give, and we create a culture of self-care and self-love that ripples out to everyone around us.

Next time you feel like brushing off your self-care routine or putting your needs at the bottom of your list, pause for a second. Think about the bigger picture. Taking time for yourself does more than just help you recharge; it sends out good vibes that touch the lives of others too. Every little thing you do to love and care for yourself makes a difference, not just for you, but for everyone around you.

Your Self-Care Toolkit: Essential Practices for Lasting Resilience

What does it really mean to take care of yourself? Well, it's different for everyone because we all have our own needs, likes, and ways of living. But there are some important things that pretty much anyone can use to build up their ability to bounce back and feel strong inside. Let's check out some of the must-haves for a solid self-care collection.

1. Mindfulness and Meditation: One of the most powerful tools for self-care and stress management is the practice of mindfulness – the simple act of bringing our attention to the present moment, without judgment or resistance. Through regular meditation or mindfulness practices, we can learn to observe our thoughts and emotions with greater clarity and equanimity, and cultivate a sense of inner peace and stability that can weather any storm.

2. Movement and Exercise: Physical activity is another essential component of self-care, not just for our bodies but also for our minds and spirits. Whether it's a gentle yoga practice, a brisk walk in nature, or a heart-pumping cardio session, regular movement helps us release tension, boost our mood and energy levels, and cultivate a greater sense of strength and resilience.

3. Nourishing Food and Hydration: The food we eat and the water we drink have a profound impact on our physical, mental, and emotional well-being. By prioritizing nourishing, whole foods and staying properly hydrated, we give our bodies the fuel and support they need to thrive, and we cultivate a greater sense of vitality and resilience from the inside out.

4. Rest and Sleep: In our fast-paced, always-on culture, it can be easy to overlook the importance of rest and sleep. But the truth is, our bodies and minds need regular periods of rest and rejuvenation in order to function at their best. By prioritizing quality sleep and building in time for rest and relaxation throughout our day, we cultivate greater resilience and the ability to show up fully in all areas of our lives.

5. Creativity and Play: Self-care isn't just about taking care of our physical needs – it's also about nurturing our minds and spirits through activities that bring us joy, creativity, and a sense of play. Whether it's engaging in a beloved hobby, trying a new art or craft, or simply letting ourselves be silly and spontaneous, regular doses of creativity and play help us cultivate greater resilience and a more joyful, fulfilling life.

6. Connection and Community: As social beings, we thrive on a sense of connection and belonging with others. By prioritizing meaningful relationships and building a supportive community around us, we cultivate greater resilience and the ability to weather life's challenges with grace and ease. This might mean scheduling regular dates with friends, joining a support group or community organization, or simply reaching out to loved ones when we need a listening ear or a helping hand.

7. Aromatherapy and the Sensory Shift Method: Last but not least, aromatherapy and the Sensory Shift Method

can be powerful additions to our self-care toolkit, helping us harness the transformative power of scent to shift our mood, release stress and tension, and cultivate greater resilience and inner strength. By incorporating specific essential oil blends and practices into our daily self-care routine, we can create a sensory anchor for the qualities and intentions we want to embody, and support ourselves in showing up as our best, most resilient selves.

Self-care really is a personal journey, you know? It's like trying out different flavors of ice cream until you find the one that makes you go, "Wow, this is it!" There's no one-size-fits-all recipe. It's all about playing around with different ideas, being kind to yourself, and believing that you'll eventually hit the jackpot with a mix that's just right for you. It's pretty exciting to think about all the options out there!

Putting it All Together: Crafting Your Empowered Self-Care Plan

So how can we put all of these pieces together into a cohesive, sustainable self-care plan? The key is to start small, be consistent, and approach self-care with a sense of intention and commitment. Here are a few tips to help you craft your own empowered self-care plan:

1. Assess your current self-care practices and identify areas for growth. Take some time to reflect on your current self-care habits and routines. What's working well? What areas could use some improvement or attention? Use this assessment as a starting point for creating your self-care plan.
2. Set clear, specific intentions for your self-care practice. What do you want to cultivate more of in your life through self-care? Greater peace and calm? More energy

and vitality? A stronger sense of self-love and self-acceptance? Get clear on your intentions, and use them as a guidepost for crafting your self-care plan.

3. Choose a few key practices to focus on, and start small. Rather than trying to overhaul your entire self-care routine overnight, choose a few key practices to focus on, and start with small, manageable steps. For example, if you want to start a daily meditation practice, begin with just 5-10 minutes a day, and gradually build up from there.

4. Create a regular self-care schedule or routine. To make self-care a consistent, non-negotiable part of your life, it can be helpful to create a regular schedule or routine. This might mean designating specific times of day for self-care practices, or building them into your existing routines (such as meditating first thing in the morning, or taking a relaxing aromatherapy bath before bed).

5. Enlist support and accountability. Self-care can be challenging, especially when we're first starting out or trying to break old patterns of self-neglect. To help stay on track and motivated, consider enlisting the support and accountability of a friend, family member, or self-care buddy. You might also consider working with a therapist, coach, or other supportive professional to help guide and support you on your self-care journey.

6. Be flexible and compassionate with yourself. Remember, self-care is not about perfection or rigidity – it's about learning to listen to and honor your own needs and desires, day by day. There will be times when life gets in the way, or when you don't feel like practicing self-care. That's okay. The key is to approach self-care with a sense of flexibility, self-compassion, and a willingness to keep showing up for yourself, no matter what.

Make sure to take a moment every now and then to see how you're doing with your self-care routine. It's okay to tweak things here and there to suit your needs better. With a bit of patience and commitment, looking after yourself will just be a regular part of your day. It'll be something that keeps you strong, bounces back from tough times, and brings happiness, helping you to be your true self in everything you do.

Conclusion: Embracing Your Resilient, Radiant Self

We're at the end of our journey with this book, and I just want to share some parting thoughts to cheer you on. It's been quite the adventure, hasn't it? We've delved into the amazing world of aromatherapy and discovered how the Sensory Shift Method can really change the game when it comes to managing stress, boosting our mood, and improving life in general. Together, we've unpacked the nuts and bolts of how scents work, mastered the craft of mixing them, and picked up a bunch of handy tips and tricks for making essential oils a part of our everyday routine.

But more than that, we've embarked on a journey of self-discovery and self-empowerment – a journey that has invited us to reconnect with our own inner wisdom, strength, and resilience. We've learned that true healing and transformation come not just from the external tools and practices we employ, but from the internal shifts and realizations that arise when we commit to nurturing and honoring ourselves on a deep, soul level.

Moving forward with your self-care and aromatherapy, I want to remind you of something important. You've got all you need inside you to grow and succeed, no matter what life throws your way. Taking care of yourself isn't being selfish—it's a deep act of loving and valuing who you are. Plus, looking after your well-being doesn't just help you; it sends out good vibes that affect everyone and everything around you.

Trust yourself as you get into aromatherapy and the Sensory Shift Method. Pay attention to what your body, heart, and soul are telling you. They'll guide you to the right practices, rituals, and scents that feel just right for you. Remember to enjoy the process and stay open to all the wonderful surprises life has to offer.

Thank you for joining me on this journey of transformation and self-discovery. It has been an honor and a privilege to share these teachings with you, and I hope that they will continue to support and inspire you as you navigate the ups and downs of life with greater ease, grace, and resilience. Know that you are not alone on this path – you are part of a global community of individuals who are committed to living with greater purpose, presence, and joy, and who are harnessing the power of self-care and natural healing to create a better world for us all.

Go ahead and let the real you shine through. Believe in the smarts and the guts you've got, and let everyone see that sparkle of yours. We're in times that could really use what only you can bring – your special touch, your kind of magic. With a little help from the scents and self-care tricks you've picked up, you're all set to face whatever comes your way. You've got this, with a heart full of courage, care for others, and a calm that won't be shaken.

With love, gratitude, and endless belief in you,
Scarlett Savage

Bibliography

Throughout the writing of this book, I have drawn upon my own extensive experience and knowledge as an aromatherapist, self-care expert, and holistic wellness practitioner. However, I have also consulted a wide range of trusted sources and reference materials to ensure the accuracy, depth, and breadth of the information presented. Below is a list of some of the key sources that have informed and inspired my work:

1. "The Complete Book of Essential Oils and Aromatherapy" by Valerie Ann Worwood - This comprehensive guide to essential oils and their therapeutic applications has been a go-to resource for me for many years, and has deeply informed my understanding of the science and art of aromatherapy.

2. "The Healing Intelligence of Essential Oils" by Kurt Schnaubelt, Ph.D. - This book offers a fascinating exploration of the chemistry and pharmacology of essential oils, as well as their role in supporting physical, emotional, and spiritual well-being.

3. "Aromatherapy: A Complete Guide to the Healing Art" by Kathi Keville and Mindy Green - This beautifully illustrated book offers a wealth of information on the history, science, and practice of aromatherapy, as well as detailed profiles of over 70 essential oils and their therapeutic properties.

4. "The Fragrant Mind: Aromatherapy for Personality, Mind, Mood, and Emotion" by Valerie Ann Worwood - This book explores the powerful connection between scent, emotion, and mental well-being, and offers practical guidance on using essential oils to support emotional balance and resilience.

5. "Aromatherapy for Healing the Spirit: Restoring Emotional and Mental Balance with Essential Oils" by Gabriel Mojay - This book offers a holistic approach to aromatherapy that incorporates principles of

traditional Chinese medicine, Ayurveda, and other healing modalities to support spiritual and emotional well-being.

6. "The Art of Blending: The Ultimate Guide to Creating Aromatic Essential Oil Blends" by Roseanne Piccirilli - This practical guide offers step-by-step instructions and creative inspiration for blending essential oils, along with detailed information on the aromatic properties and therapeutic benefits of over 100 essential oils.

7. "Essential Oils in Spiritual Practice: Working with the Chakras, Divine Archetypes, and the Five Great Elements" by Candice Covington - This book explores the use of essential oils in spiritual and energetic healing practices, and offers guidance on creating custom blends for meditation, prayer, and ritual.

8. "The Essential Oils Hormone Solution" by Dr. Mariza Snyder - This book offers a groundbreaking approach to using essential oils to balance hormones, reduce stress, and support women's health and well-being at every stage of life.

9. "The Ultimate Guide to Aromatherapy" by Jade Shutes and Amy Galper - This comprehensive guide offers a wealth of information on the history, science, and practice of aromatherapy, as well as detailed profiles of over 50 essential oils and their therapeutic properties.

10. "Aromatherapy for Beginners: The Complete Guide to Getting Started with Essential Oils" by Anne Kennedy - This beginner-friendly guide offers a clear and concise introduction to the world of aromatherapy, with practical tips and techniques for using essential oils safely and effectively.

These are just a few of the many trusted sources that have informed my work as an aromatherapist and self-care expert. I am deeply grateful to the many teachers, mentors, and colleagues who have shared their wisdom and knowledge with me over the years, and I hope that this book will serve as a valuable resource and guide for anyone seeking to harness the transformative power of essential oils and aromatherapy in their own lives.

www.ingramcontent.com/pod-product-compliance
Lightning Source LLC
Chambersburg PA
CBHW051913250726
48659CB00002B/627